AF348570

WELL, THAT WAS STRANGE

ACKNOWLEDGEMENTS

Writing my story was one of the most emotional, challenging, and rewarding experiences of my life. I began writing this four years ago when I first started dealing with severe mental health challenges. I would like to thank my amazing family, very best friends, non-biological sisters, and colleagues for supporting me during this process. This wouldn't have been possible without you. Thank you for believing in me.

- Bailey, Bails, Bai

xoxo

WELL, THAT WAS STRANGE

A TRUE STORY ABOUT A YOUNG ADULT WHO LEARNED TO LIVE WITH MANIC PSYCHOSIS

BAILEY EMILY

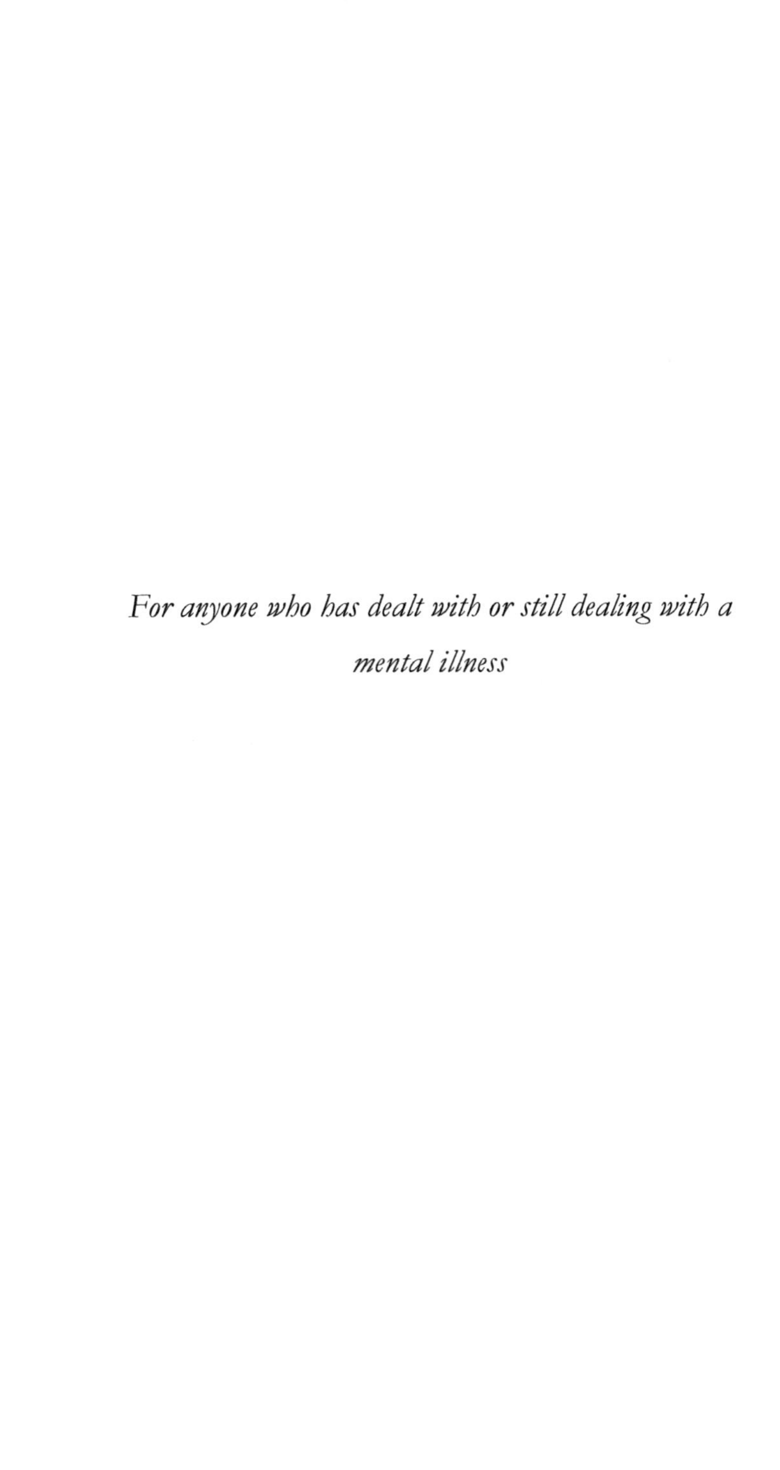

For anyone who has dealt with or still dealing with a mental illness

CONTENTS

PREFACE

I am writing this because manic psychosis changed my life completely. It has taught me the power of healing, courage, and, most importantly, how to be a better advocate for those dealing with mental health obstacles.

Manic psychosis is something that I'll never shut up about; why? Well, it affects more people than we think. It's a scary illness, and it took a lot of resilience and strength to get to where I am today.

I felt inspired to add to the book I began writing back in June of 2019. Most of what I wrote was written as I was experiencing my lengthy manic episode. The "visions" (as I used to call them) that I experienced while writing were hallucinations.

The scary part about manic psychosis is that I thought the hallucinations were real. It took time, but I healed, and I am no longer in a manic state. They say that "time heals everything." Does it? It definitely can, at least with most things.

I realized not long after my episode, with the help of professionals, that what I was experiencing was in fact, manic psychosis. My family and I had never heard of it. That's another reason why I'm writing this. There needs to be more awareness on this topic.

A couple of years ago, I made the difficult decision to write a new blog post entitled; "My Experience with Psychosis." I was holding this in for so long. Was it challenging? Of course, but I knew it was time. I was afraid of what others would think of me. Would they think I was weird? Different? Scary? Many thoughts began to race through my head.

Most of my close friends and family knew what had happened to me; however, a lot of people had no idea. Clicking the share button had my whole body heating up with anxiety. After I received such kind and supportive feedback…I felt free. The people that I have in my life mean everything to me.

Sometimes it can be scary to envision what you might have to do to bounce back from a mental illness like this/explain it to others. I am here to tell you that you don't have to until you're ready…or you don't have to at all.

A huge goal of mine has always been to publish my own book. I decided to write this to spread awareness and educate others. I feel as though psychosis can be a topic that not a lot of people understand, and that's okay! In all honesty, I don't think it's talked about enough, considering how many people go through this. I hope I can at least try my best to put the puzzle pieces together for you.

After sharing my blog post, I realized that you should never be ashamed of your mental illness. For the longest time, I was embarrassed about what had happened to me. The psychosis illness is some scary stuff, but it has made me a stronger person. It has taught me more life lessons than I could have ever imagined at such a young age.

I was able to discover a lot of my own interests and become educated on this topic. Most importantly, it has given me the strength to help others.

I know first-hand what dealing with a mental illness is like, so I would never want anyone to go through what I went through without help and support.

Before you begin reading my story, I'd like to say this; you can 100% "grow through what you go through" (Gibson, 2023), and yes, there's almost always a light at the end of the tunnel, even if it seems impossible. Life has a way of testing our limits and presenting us with unfortunate circumstances. I'm here to tell you that it can get better. Trust me.

UNANSWERED QUESTIONS

Saturday July 20th, 2019

As I lay here on a rainy, calm, Saturday evening, with a goji berry-scented hair mask marinating in my hair; I have a lot on my mind. How did this happen to me? How will I heal? Does it get better? Will the meds work? It's frustrating because I don't know the answers. On a more positive note, I had a nice conversation with my grandma last night. She picked me up at about 12:30 a.m. from my best friend's surprise party. I explained to my grandma how I believed I was different from all my friends. I told her that what's been going on makes me feel upset from time to time. I know that this is my thing, and it's manageable, but it's hard.

My grandma tried to give me advice. It's got to be difficult unless you are facing a mental illness yourself, which she is not. She said to me that my brain is okay. I thought that I needed a neuroscientist to get in there weeks ago.

She said, "Imagine that your brain is wired, and something may just not be connected properly, and that is okay." I felt at peace once she told me that. What I went through weeks ago has turned me into a new individual. It was a scary turn of events.

THE BEGINNING OF IT ALL

September 2018

Present me: First-year university was difficult for me. I was a homebody, and leaving my job, friends, and family made my heart drop completely. I spent so much time battling my depression. I understand that many teens deal with this first year of university, and I feel for them; I do, but don't worry, it can get better!

I tried my best to pull it together, but I just couldn't get there. The fact that I was trying so hard was horrible when it came to my mental health and self-care routines. I went through university in tears almost every day; however, I had all the support I could have asked for. I was surrounded by my family members, very best friends, colleagues, my don, my universities dance team, help from their mental health resources, one of my roommates (a complete angel), and of course one of my closest friends (also my roommate) who was there for me every step of the way.

She saw me at my worst and never gave up. She wanted what was best for me and wanted me to heal. I'll never forget that. My goal is to treat others the way she treated me. I'm never going to stop trying to help somebody that needs me. She taught me that.

Bailey – August 2019: The number of times I said I was going to drop out of school was insane, and thanks for everyone's support because I'm glad I stayed too. **Present me:** I dropped out two months into my second year, unfortunately.

Even though what I went through is something that I would never, ever wish upon anyone, it turned me into a new and stronger individual who I'm kind of vibing with. I feel like I have grown up and can look at the world differently. Maybe from a more mature point of view, if you will. I like that about me!

During my first semester of university, I was extremely depressed. Nothing could have persuaded me to leave my bed. I didn't go out, I stayed in, cleaned, did homework, and that's about it. It's weird because I was so outgoing and always on the go.

One of my best friends came over religiously to put a smile on my face. She always succeeded and knew exactly how to make me laugh. Her frequent visits to my student apartment were the only moments I would laugh that day instead of cry. Sounds sad, but it's the truth. I love her.

My best friend (roommate) and I used to plan our lives while drinking coffee from our Keurig. We would have constant life chats with our other amazing roommate as we watched **This Is Us** every Tuesday when we could.

Friends and family are so important to surround yourself with. Sometimes it can even be the answer to a lot of your own issues! It has truly helped me out in so many cases. When I came home for Thanksgiving, Christmas, and literally every single weekend, my family would constantly ask me if I was okay. I told them I was sad but had no further details. I wish I had told them, but I felt like I would be letting people down. I didn't want to give up. School was so important to me.

I know it sounds dramatic, but when my dad picked me up every weekend, I felt like being home was like entering a new world. A world of peace and hope for something better to come along.

Second semester was a lot better! My best friend and I joined a club, and I joined the dance team. She and my other roommate decided to work out; we ate a lot of burrito bowls, laughed, and kept it cool. Overall, I felt 100% better than how I was feeling before. It was priceless. I was suffering for an entire semester. As soon as I was starting to feel like myself again, it was like a breath of fresh air. It's crazy how life can fall into place so unexpectedly.

Leading up to university, I was different. I was losing my spark. I didn't want to leave what I had in the small city I grew up in. I was nervous about going away, and always had the idea in my mind of taking a year off. This was not because I needed time to consider my program. This was simply because, I wanted to put off the idea of going to school for as long as I could.

Leading up to a few days before move-in, as I left my friends, family, and job, I felt like there was a hole in my heart. I wasn't happy, and I knew it. If you know me well, you know I'm almost always happy; at least, I try to be. I love to chat, laugh, sing, and dance. I enjoy cute little coffee dates, going to my favourite restaurants, conversing with anyone and everyone, and Marshall's. It's sad because, at this time I felt like I had nothing at all. I felt lost.

Bailey – August 2019: This evening as I write, I'm not lost, and I'm happier and getting better. I'm a new person who can't wait to go back to school. I also have the opportunity to be a part of a fantastic team there! I can't wait to see what the future holds and what my degree will lead me to!

A SCARY FEW WEEKS

My Manic Episode

June 2019

Something happened almost a month ago that was completely unexpected. I was driving down a street in my city with a very close friend of mine. I got into a minor car accident. We're okay, but I was mad at myself. I hit someone who was probably driving home from work on a normal day, and not to mention with precious cargo in my vehicle.

I felt broken for weeks. I had a lot going on, and this threw me over the edge. I was in tears one night, about a week after the accident. I faced severe trauma from what had happened, even though we were completely okay. I couldn't stop the "what ifs" from spiraling in my head. It felt impossible. I wanted to talk it through with the friend I had gotten into the accident with; she was all ears and so much help on the other line. I just love her!

Just days after, something more serious happened. This time I was up from 7 pm-almost 9 am. My mom, dad, grandma, aunt, one of gram's best friends, my stepdad, and stepmom were worried out of their minds. They had every right to be.

I was on Facetime with my aunt at five in the morning when I self-diagnosed myself with PTSD (Wasn't an accurate diagnosis).

Present me: Disclaimer - The next part of my story is where it gets a little, well…interesting, I guess. Not really sure what word to use. I contemplated even putting this part in my book, but I know it's important. This was out of the norm, frightening, and incredibly shocking. I want to tell you because this is something that not only, I have dealt with, but many others who have experienced a manic episode. I want people to know what actually happens.

Suddenly, out of nowhere, clear hallucinations of my passing loved ones appeared in my room. My great grandma drifted into my room like a kite. She immediately made me jump. I could see her. Her silhouette was clear as day. I'm talking like physically being able to see facial features. Yep, insane, I know. I was speaking a mile a minute as she tapped me lightly on my feet, then on my waist.

After this happened, one of gram's best friend's (Char) went to work, and so did gram. Char was the first person to witness all of this. She didn't freak out; she just sat with me. She's simply the best.

My family refused to leave me alone. My mom rushed over and came to lay with me in my bed. Seconds later, one of my favourite mascaras drifted out of my drawer. I jumped.

My mom laid in bed with me and tried her best to get me to sleep. It was almost impossible because the hallucinations wouldn't stop. My mom was on the phone with the Mental Health Association when this was happening. I had no clue who she was talking to; however, she told me later, and I'm glad she called.

Several hallucinations occurred where I could feel five senses of my loved ones in my bedroom. My grandparents on my dad's side appeared right after my great grandmother. I could feel my grandparents (like physically being able to hear, see, and feel them).

My grandma was at work when all of this was happening, but seconds later, she was on her way home to be with me. I freaked out as soon as I saw a moving image of her silhouette floating into my room.

She was wearing my dad's Olympics zip-up hoodie. I cried even harder when I saw her silhouette flash brightly before my eyes and into a dark fog. I thought she was on her way home and had gotten into a car accident. Weird assumption, I know.

I cried and told my mom to get a hold of her and ensure that she was okay. She was. After asking my great grandma to sing one of her favourite songs Singin' in the Rain by Gene Kelly, she did, I heard it, and I flipped out. I began to cough and could feel a lukewarm Campbell's soup going down my throat as my dad's mom stirred me tea.

One of the last hallucinations I experienced that day was my grandma's passing husband. He passed away right before I was born from cancer. It started in the lungs and then moved to his brain.

Naturally, I only ever saw him in pictures and old videos here and there. The one thing I do know is that he made my grandma the happiest woman on the planet. I know he had to have been a great man.

He drifted from the side of my bed wearing a hat, jeans, and a flannel. I saw him with a cigarette in hand, and my mom tried to see him too. When she looked at him (not able to see anything, obviously), he flipped around as if he wasn't smoking. **Present me:** Yes, it was terrifying, but I guess it proves how interesting the brain can be.

After texting and "Instagram-storying" people about this, my mom deleted some of the stuff I put on my story. Thank God she did that…those posts were crazy.

The only two things I kept repeating all day was that I wanted to hang out with my friends, and close at work that day. Makes sense.

Days after, I had another episode, small compared to the first one. I was adamant about having someone there for the first week and a half because it made me feel protected.

That night my grandma slept in my bed with me, and I could feel the presence of my great grandma and my grandma's husband in my room.

Three things severely frightened me as a kid: Thunder, lightning, and fireworks. I was afraid of anything that was loud and abrupt. Nine times out of ten, I would run to my grandma's bed on a noisy rainy night. As she would try to console me, she used to say this; "Let's climb up on our ladder up to the moon, and that thunder you're hearing, that's just the angels bowling."

During my episode, there was a torrential downpour and lightning. I panicked. I was having another episode, and so I went into my fanny pack. (**Present me**: Anytime I had an episode, I would grab a pen and paper and write about what I was seeing.) I didn't grab a pen because I would have woken up my grandma from climbing over her.

Instead, I grabbed my expensive Kylie Jenner

liquid lipstick and started to write in an old Cosmopolitan magazine. Classic. As we talked about this a few days later, gram and Char said, "Don't you know you wrote that book backwards?" I laughed and said, "yeah, right."

I did. It was crazy because everything I wrote in that magazine made sense to me. My grandma and Char had no idea what I was writing about. They read it but couldn't grasp the story I was trying to tell, obviously.

Present me: I bet you if I found that magazine today, I would have no idea what it said. That's the scariest part of psychosis. Everything that once made sense is a blur as soon as the episode ends. After my intense manic episode, I went to seek medical attention from my family doctor that morning. I was not hospitalized, as the hallucinations were rather pleasant compared to the ones others have encountered. Also, my family refused to put me in a psych ward. They didn't believe it was fair to leave me there. Instead, they watched over me and tried their best to understand. I am very lucky. I was also not putting myself or others in danger. My whole family came. (It's like that part in My Big Fat Greek Wedding where the entire Greek family drops their daughter, niece, granddaughter off at college.)

Present me: My family did everything for me during this time. They put their lives on hold to make sure that I was okay. Each of them had shifts to come and be with me, whether that meant staying the night, hanging out with me all day, or taking me to Indigo or Marshall's. I could not be alone, and they refused to let me suffer. I love my family so much and will continue to appreciate what they did for me during such a difficult time in my life.

I remember so vividly the day after my first episode. My whole family came over, and they dropped everything. My mom and aunt took me to all-you-can-eat sushi, and we walked along the water later that afternoon. Immediately after, they took me to Indigo so that I could buy more pens to use for my journal.

If I remember correctly, my aunt went back home to Toronto to grab some stuff because she had been staying with me that whole time. She came back with fun new stationary things. I was in awe as I stared at all these boujee pastel highlighters and cool pens. It was like my eyes were going to turn into heart shapes. It was such a kind gesture.

My dad and stepmom also stayed by my side for all of it, as did my grandma and Char. I knew they didn't want to see me like this, so it was time for me to receive help asap. I also didn't have a choice. All three of my younger sisters would come over to swim, so it was a peaceful couple of weeks, although it was scary. As I said before, it's crazy how somebody's brain can even do such a thing. I never thought it would be me. I remember taking a blood and urine test to prove that I was not on hard drugs.

Honestly, I don't blame people for thinking I was on drugs based on how I was acting. My energy was at an all-time high; I was speaking a mile a minute, and every connection I explained and the "visions" I encountered made no sense at all. Now I understand why. I was telling people that this was almost some kind of hidden talent/ability which was honestly what I thought. What I was experiencing was in fact; manic psychosis, and the crazy part was that I had no idea. I didn't realize that the things I was connecting to my life, including characters from television shows and movies, were coincidences… and for me, that is the scariest part of psychosis.

I remember the day that my best friends came over to see me. I was only allowed to have certain people come and visit. They are some of the most important people in my life, and I love them so much. I was saying some crazy stuff, and nothing made sense, but to me, it seemed like it did. Everyone else was confused…No s***. I don't blame them.

I remember telling them that we would all be on The Ellen Show because of my cool abilities, so looking back on it, I can't help but laugh! I love my best friends because they have accepted me for who I am and always will. They watched me go through something so frightening. Despite the insane stuff that occurred, they never left my side. That's what friends do, and they have never once failed. We'll be together till the end.

My roommate/best friend was coming over frequently to see me. She was working three hours away, and still managed to come and be with me. She brought me journals, activities, and pens. She wanted to make sure I would be okay, and it showed. She is honestly a one in a million and will always hold a special place in my heart.

I spoke to my doctor about what I was experiencing one on one. She was all ears. I told her everything, and we collectively agreed that I needed a lot of help. I received it immediately and was referred to a program at my nearest hospital.

This program is an early intervention service for anyone that has experienced their first episode of psychosis. I'm glad I got the help. I met some of the most kind and supportive individuals/therapists ever! Each of them has incredible powers, and in all honesty, they saved me. Not only was I working with multiple therapists, but I was also introduced to a great psychiatrist. He was able to help me understand what I was going through from point A to Z. I believe I was diagnosed with psychosis and bipolar disorder. (To be honest, I still don't really know my diagnosis.)

When you piece that together it can be classified as manic psychosis. Psychosis can occur after an individual has experienced a long depressive episode. If they start to have intense feelings of euphoria this can turn into a bipolar episode.

For me, the extreme mood swings from long-term depression to sudden changes in lifestyle and euphoric thoughts triggered a breakdown. That's how I believe it happened, but even with the help of professionals, it's hard to be sure.

When I read more into it, everything began to click. According to CAMH, "The word psychosis is used to describe conditions that affect the mind, in which people have trouble distinguishing between what is real and what is not" (CAMH, 2023).

When an individual is experiencing psychosis, they may experience delusions and hallucinations that could be auditory or visual. I'm being 100% honest when I say that I experienced every one of those symptoms, and let me tell you, it was freaky.

I went and am still going to therapy. After my first episode, I started taking medication for the first time. I was on an anti-psychotic drug, which made me want to eat six junior chickens in one sitting, but it worked, so I didn't care.

I took a mental health break from everything and was without electronics for almost three weeks. Although I felt deprived of social media as many other 18-year-olds would, I was able to clear my head from everything I saw online. I would recommend everyone to try it if they can.

I took time for myself, and every single person was supportive. I am so thankful that I'm surrounded by so many amazing individuals. This is manic

psychosis, and THE SUPPORT IS INSANE.

A PORTUGUESE FESTA

August 2019

My Aunt comes down from California once or twice a year! When she arrives my family and I spend tons of time with her! After my grandfather (avô) and my grandmother (avó) passed away, my family and I made it a tradition to have a Portuguese festa. It's a yearly barbecue where we chat, laugh, dance, make "spritada" (basically beef on a stick), eat carbs, play games, and spend quality time together. I look forward to this barbeque every year, except this time, it was different. I was having these "visions" of my passing loved ones in my room just days prior. My parents felt like I would be overwhelmed when I went. This is because they knew what would happen. They knew it would be possible for me to have another breakdown.

My stepmom and her mom picked me up from my house at around 4 o'clock. The rest of my family was already at the barbecue. When they picked me up, I brought a journal that I was writing at the time. It had way too many details in it. I'll leave it at that. Thanks to my stepmom for convincing me to leave it in the car. Love you for that; it was a lot.

I was in the car with my stepmom and her mom, rehearsing how I would walk through those gates. I lunged over my sister's car seat and onto the concrete. My stepmom said, "Remember, these Portuguese people can be a little emotional at times." She's not wrong, so I walked through those gates as if everything was normal, or at least I tried. At this point, the only people that knew about this were my dad, stepmom, my stepmom's mom, my aunts, my uncle, my cousin, and her husband (I have a big family). My stepmom, my dad, and I had a special code. If my "visions" appeared, I would lower my new sunglasses onto the bridge of my nose. Useful trick.

Just as we thought, I was starting to have a few "visions". These hallucinations were visual, not auditory, or sensory, of my grandparents all around this sunny backyard covered in colourful coral, teal, and bright blue summer decor. I tried my best to ignore what I saw but it was near impossible. I was positive I would hallucinate, so I was prepared. Not only was I prepared for the "visions", but I was ready to tell more family members later that evening. Before dropping the news on everyone else, I told my closest cousins first. **Present me:** Keep in mind that I was telling family and friends I had some sort of a talent or ability, not knowing that I was going through psychosis.

It was so hard to keep it from the rest of my family, but I didn't want to put a damper on the birthday celebration we were having for my aunt. It's okay; if you guys read this, you'll all know now, and I can't wait to start talking about it more.

At around 7 o'clock I told two more of my sweet cousins. They just sat and listened. I told them everything and explained that "I can stop whenever if this is a lot." They just listened. I love them so much, and I'm glad they were so chill about the situation. My cousin jumped out of her boyfriend's truck when she was leaving. I ran towards her, jumped into her arms,

and told her I loved her. She said she loved me too.

MY DIAGNOSIS

I went to receive help from specialists and was diagnosed. I was diagnosed with manic psychosis. As I said before, this is basically a mixture of psychosis and bipolar disorder (I believe).

It wasn't easy to deal with at first. I felt like even my family and closest friends couldn't understand me, and that's okay; it's probably hard to understand me sometimes. It's all good though; this is my thing, and it's manageable.

I've done a lot of healing since then, and I am getting better at accepting that this is a part of me. We all have issues and things going on! Although our battles may differ from our friends and family…we're all going through something. That is why it's important to check in on your loved ones, simply because you never know what someone could be experiencing.

I'm currently on medication to combat the manic episodes. (**Present me:** This was the first anti-psychotic drug I started taking.) I take one half during the day and a full at night.

Yes, I do get bloated, and have gained weight, but it's working right now. I did try to wean myself off the daily dose without discretion. That was a mistake. You know what, it wasn't though, because I realized what would happen if I did go off the meds right now. Lesson learned.

I will be moving towards a newer medication soon. One of my close friends helped me understand the whole medication thing. She said that she had to go on many different types of medications to find out what was best for her, and I believe it. On August 1st, mine should be switched. Meds can be tricky and not always everyone's cup of tea, but for me, it has helped so much.

BODY IMAGE

Medication is something that has changed my body a lot. I'm a 22-year-old female, so my body is constantly changing, but this was more than that. It was affecting me, and it wouldn't stop.

I've never been one to have issues with my body, but ever since I began taking medication, I was gaining a lot more weight. I'm not going to sugar-coat it; I was insecure, and I knew it. As I said before, immediately after I experienced manic psychosis, I started taking my first dose of medication. Although it does combat the side effects of psychosis, one thing that it did do, however, was increase my appetite.

For me, it wasn't just a little bit; it was a lot. I went through high school with a relatively healthy lifestyle. I was a competitive dancer, and at the time, it was my whole life. I was so passionate about it. Dancing helped relieve any of my stress.

I worked as many shifts as possible, achieved high grades, and ate…well, okay. Since I was dancing almost every day of the week for hours on end, I ate a lot of red meat and vegetables.

Anyways, my point is that when I was in my worst state of depression just months after my manic episode and leaving university, two things happened. I was allowing the medication to take over my life, as well as my eating habits.

Keep in mind that it was the first round of Covid lockdowns, so I ordered take-out at least 2-3 times a week. I was literally addicted. I craved everything and anything while on this medication. It was strange because when I was gaining weight, I didn't even realize. Looking back on it, I don't think it was because I didn't realize, it was simply because I was too depressed to care.

I gained 25-30 lbs. When I went back to work that summer after the lengthy Covid lockdown, I felt as though I looked like a completely different person. That's when I started to care. My mood was increasing so, therefore, I was beginning to question why I looked the way I did.

I ended up going off this medication. Like I said before, it's all about trial and error. Meds can be difficult. Be patient though, they could really help you, although I understand that they're not for everybody.

I'm finally pretty happy in my own skin. I lost most of the weight in a healthy way by walking and ordering less take-out. I'm not really a gym kind of a girl so I enjoy going on long walks!

Do what's right for you, and always try your best to take care of your body! You only get one. It's never too late to start making changes to your lifestyle!

SYMPTOMS

In terms of my symptoms, I had many. After I overcame my major manic episode, I researched the common symptoms. I needed to know what was happening to my brain, so I took the time to figure it out.

One of the symptoms of psychosis is hallucinations. During an episode; seeing, hearing, and feeling things that aren't there can be possible. Crazy, I know, but this is something that I had to deal with. It could literally happen to anybody.

Overspending is another big one. When I was going through psychosis, I spent thousands of dollars at Indigo and Marshalls. I mean, don't get me wrong, I love a little retail therapy, but this was excessive. I was also not in the right state of mind.

Next is high energy. Sometimes it's hard to differentiate between my manic high energy and my "non-manic" high energy. I'm already a super energetic individual. However, when I'm manic, it's out of the norm. During my manic state, I was talking a mile a minute. Additionally, I would always be thinking about a million things at once.

My brain was filled to the brim with tasks, creative ideas, conversations I would have with my friends and family, connections…It didn't stop.

Creativity was another one of my symptoms, even though I've always been a creative individual. Growing up, my dad was an art teacher, so art was something that I was constantly surrounded by as a kid. I loved it. I've always been into drawing and painting from the very beginning; it's still a big part of my life today. I was a shy kid in my first couple of years in elementary school. When I didn't want to play with the other kids at recess, I would sit in the corner, leaned against a brick wall, and draw in my sketchbook. I would be so excited to get home and show my family my drawings of the day. Sorry, off-topic.

Anyways, when I was in my manic state, I was slightly more creative than usual. I could paint anything I envisioned in my head, and it would be picture-perfect. Wild. Although what I went through was spine-chilling, this was definitely the "cooler" part of psychosis. The last symptom that I will be talking about is the connections. This symptom affected me the most. When somebody is going through psychosis, they may start connecting things to their life that aren't necessarily true.

I would start to connect my life to certain characters in tv shows. Friends was a big one. Things that would happen in the plot, or phrases the characters would say, somehow made me think that everything was connected to me. Now that I think about it, I didn't know that my brain was capable of doing such a thing. I know I keep saying that, but it's true.

Another thing that I did was write all my connections in a journal. I can't explain this part because I don't even understand what I was doing. As I said before, I looked in that journal a couple of weeks ago and didn't understand a thing. So, there's that. The most embarrassing one by far was all the Instagram stories. I don't even like bringing this up. I was posting stuff that I was sure connected to me somehow. It did not.

When I was in my manic state, I was positive that it did. Manic psychosis is frightening, although it kind of proves how amazing the brain can be. How did my brain do that? I'll never be sure.

LOSING MY IDENTITY

52

When I was going through manic psychosis, I lost myself. I didn't know who I was or what I was doing. It's funny though because at the time, I thought that manic psychosis was so cool.

I was going around telling all my close friends and family that this was my gift. This mental disorder I was dealing with made me believe that I had cool abilities. It made me think that I was different.

Looking back on it, I don't remember much of what I was doing or saying. To this day, I still have friends and family telling me about all the things I said while going manic. Thank God most of those phrases were funny.

When I was going through manic psychosis, I wasn't myself. It was like my soul literally left my body. That eighteen-year-old girl who thought she had extraordinary psychic abilities was not me. I know that now. Sometimes I think about what I went through and can't help but cry. I look back and wonder how I didn't realize that everything was connections and coincidences.

Sometimes I beat myself up, but I need to remember that this was something that happened to my brain. It was out of my control, and I never saw any of this coming. It happened, and that's just it.

Psychosis has the power to make people lose their identity. Truthfully, I can't even explain how I felt. Afraid, maybe? I guess I'll leave it at that.

THE BOOK

So, remember that book I was talking about earlier? Well, now I'm here to talk about the nitty gritty, the ins and outs, the embarrassing, weird, and cringey journal entries. I started the journal because my best friend bought it for me. The whole point was to write down what I was going through; however, I took it to the extremes.

I had just gotten into a car accident with one of my "non-biological sisters," so I was beating myself up. One of my first journal entries was for her. I was writing to get over what had happened and to apologize. I was lucky because she forgave me from the moment it happened. That's how amazing she is. She didn't want me to be upset.

Besides the accident, I had a lot going on mentally, and I was starting to turn to alcohol, partying, plus I was barely sleeping. That only lasted for a week, but it had a significantly negative impact on my life.

The interesting part about all of this was that I was getting symptoms of psychosis days before my major manic episode. My energy was at an all-time high, and I felt like I was sensing things.

The connections were also starting. Yeah, it was wild. This was about a week or so after some of my worst days. As I was experiencing those symptoms, I went out for coffee with another one of my "non-biological sisters".

What I love the most about her was this; I told her everything, was clearly going a little bonkers, and she never looked at me differently. She listened and gave me a lot of advice. One of the third or fourth journal entries was about her.

If you knew me during this time, you knew that I had taken that book everywhere. I wasn't going to stop writing until it was full. I was having a lot of issues, so as you can imagine; it filled up quick. It started with regular journal entries, but as soon as I became more manic, they got rather detailed. Not only that, but they weren't making much sense to anyone but me.

I'd open the journal now to get a better idea, but I physically cannot. I quickly flipped through it a week or so ago. I got really emotional. It takes me back to those times, and it scares me. It makes me think about the person I was when I was going manic. I wasn't a bad person if anything, I was funnier…but it wasn't me.

When I had my hallucinations, I used the book to document all of it. I wrote about everything I saw and didn't leave out one detail. That journal helped me write this book.

All the hallucinations I told you about were taken directly from those journal entries. I wrote my journal entry about my "visions" on June 19th, 2019. That was the day of my major manic episode. After all the hallucination entries came the connections. Many of the connections I wrote were about the people in my life.

Before I had my phone taken away (for my own good), I was scrolling through Instagram quite frequently. I would see certain posts and think they somehow had to do with me. Yeah, I'm just as confused as you are.

After my phone was taken away, I had no choice but to watch Netflix all day. My obsession with Friends was real. I thought that I was just like Phoebe Buffay. She was the cool one with good vibes, so I wanted to be like her too, and thought I was similar. Even certain things that would happen in the plot had me connecting it to my own life.

I honestly can't believe I'm talking about this publicly because I was super embarrassed for the longest time. I've come to learn that this happened to me, and I'm just going to accept it. I want to be honest with everyone, and I'm not going to cover it up anymore. Like I said before, this could happen to anyone. I'm proud of myself for having the courage to share what I went through personally. The point is to make someone else feel like they are not alone, and I hope I can do that.

PERSPECTIVES

When I was going through manic psychosis/dealing with minor symptoms years after, I was not in the right head space; therefore, I didn't know what was happening to me. I had some of my close friends and family write about how they felt when I was dealing with this mental illness. How did they view me? What was going through their minds? It was interesting to look at it from their perspective.

Grandma – Jackie Eager

The morning of Bailey's psychosis started out like any other morning for me, up at 5 AM getting ready for work. I could hear Bailey talking to someone, and then she was talking to me, and I said, "Bails, I have to get ready for work, and why are you up so early?"

You have to realize we knew nothing about what was going on. I thought Bailey was just being Bailey, a bit hyper and feeling super chatty. I felt so bad now that I left for work and left her like that.

Jenna called me once I was at work and said, "Mom, something is wrong with Bailey. She is talking to Murray and Nanny and seems too not be herself." I called Lisa (Bailey's Mom) and relayed what Jenna had said. Lisa rushed over and called me to say, "Mom, something is not right." I rushed home to find Bailey talking to Murray and Nan, both who had passed away. For the next few days and nights, we sat with Bailey, never leaving her alone. She would say, "Gram, Murray is in the corner Nanny is here! I love them, but I'm scared. Make them go away." Out the sage would come. I saged maybe fifteen times a night, and only then would she go to sleep.

One night as I was sitting with her, she showed me what she wrote and read to me what she was feeling. I looked at her writing, and it was just letters that made no sense to anyone but Bailey.

I remember going into the bathroom sobbing. I was so scared. Here was my Granddaughter, the light of my life, going through something, and I had no idea how to help her. The only thing we could do was be there for her until we could get some clarity as to what was happening and get help. We called all the helplines, and there was no help. Zero help. It was so scary. Lisa can fill in the blanks on getting the help that was needed. After we did get help.

I remember Bailey saying, "Gram, what if I am never normal again?" and I said, "Bails, what is normal? You are normal, just a different kind of normal."

I hope when she writes her book; it helps others to realize you can overcome your old norm and embrace your new normal. I still cry sometimes when I think of what happened, and still have no idea how this happened to a bright, "normal" young person.

What I do know is that I am grateful for this beautiful young person who fills all our lives with joy, and yep, she still talks 90 miles an hour…but that's our Bailey, and I would not change one thing about her.

Mom – Lisa Eager

If you know Bailey, you know she's full of life, positive, always happy, and never stops talking! She is the life of the party and the girl who cherishes her family and friends! She is loved by everyone she meets! Beautiful, talented, extremely intelligent, funny, and the kind of person that just makes you feel good!

I will never forget when Bailey turned eighteen! That year she had applied to all kinds of universities thrilled to start her new life away from home. Little did we know she was struggling and feeling a new fear of leaving her life at home behind. To her it felt like everything was falling apart. We assured her it's normal to feel this way and that the first year is always difficult. Home was also not that far away.

We spent the summer getting her ready for uni and helping her decorate her new apartment in residence! It was such an exciting time, but I slowly started to watch my happy girl become someone else, a new sad version of my once cheerful girl. I assured her this would pass but it continued to get worse. I wish I realized she was slipping away into severe depression, but I really just thought it was the first-year blues and it would soon pass.

That summer after first year Bailey came home and she wasn't the same cheerful and full of life girl. She was sad, depressed, and so down. It crushed my heart. I remember picking her up from work during summer break and she was not at all herself. It wasn't uncommon for Bailey to talk and chat, however, there was something very unusual about the way she was speaking. I remember talking to my mom after dropping her off. She also felt like something was off.

The next morning all our lives shifted. I remember a call from my mom and my sister telling me, "Lisa, something is wrong with Bailey!" I called into work and rushed to make sure she was okay. What happened next was so frightening. I ran into her room, she was hallucinating, and she was talking to my grandmother who had passed a few years ago. She was laying in her bed giving me graphic details of our family that had passed away.

She believed she was a psychic and sharing things with our loved ones who had passed. She was telling me my grandmother was right over in the corner chatting with her and that my stepdad was also beside her, and she was describing him exactly as he was. "Do you see them, mom?" Those words literally still sit in my mind. I didn't know what was happening, I grabbed her tightly and laid in her bed holding her telling her everything is okay.

I was completely terrified of what was happening! Was she doing drugs? I felt fear strike through me as I asked her what she had taken? She said, "Mom, nothing…I haven't taken anything." I thought to myself was she okay!!? Was she scared? She didn't know anything that was going on! I continued to hold her until more family came. I called several places for help and unfortunately, there was none! No one could help! I called and called, and I refused to take no for an answer. I wasn't going to take her to any hospital as I knew I could figure this out on my own until I pretty much couldn't. I asked her questions, and I finally called our family physician for help and begged them to see her.

We took her in that morning, and after some testing, the doctor confirmed she was having a manic episode. The only time I ever heard of this was in my university psych textbook, and of course, it was nothing like what I was actually witnessing. There was no way, I thought.

Our doctor confirmed that due to the depression she had been experiencing, her brain had switched into a full-on manic episode. I can't tell you how difficult it was for me to get answers that morning and I had to fight for Bailey, and I wouldn't stop until I knew what to do. Our family doctor put in a referral later that day. After many phone calls, we met with a psychologist at the hospital, who confirmed she was experiencing early psychosis. It was shockingly common during first-year stress from school, life changes, or other stressful events. I knew we needed to do everything to keep her, and I did everything in my power to educate myself on what was happening to her. It was one of the most painful, eye-opening, scary times of our lives. To see your child fall apart before your eyes is devastating.

Over the next couple of days, with the help of incredible family and friends and the hospital program, we were able to learn more and more. How scary is it to see someone's mind alter the way hers did. One day you are yourself; the next day, your mind switches on you and you completely lose touch of reality.

That week I tried to shelter her from the world as I was still learning about what was happening. I was afraid and wanted her to be stress-free. If this were to happen again, I would now know what to do. At that time, I was an absolute mess trying to hold it all in. My family and I wanted to make sure she was okay and to get whatever help we could.

Bailey's friends were reaching out and were concerned. A part of me was afraid for them to see her this way. I wondered how she would react or how they would react to what was happening.

If I can say one thing, Bailey has the biggest support group I have ever seen! Her lifelong friends were there for her and saw her go through this, as scary and confusing as it was. If anything, they loved her even more. Our family and friends took shifts to be with her, so she wasn't alone during the day.

The amount of support we had was nothing I ever expected, and we wouldn't have gotten through it without them.

During Bailey's breakdown, she was writing journal entries. She was writing upside down and could read it perfectly. Suddenly these journals became the only thing she talked about. It made no sense to anyone but her, and as I sat there listening to these entries, I remember holding back tears until I couldn't take it anymore.

I would go into my car and cry and cry. How could this happen to her? How can your own brain do this to you? Will she ever be the Bailey we always knew? Would she get through it? Would she be okay? Questions just flooded through my head.

That week I used all the resources given to me and met with family members of others who had been through this. I reached out to a pharmacist I worked with who said he sees this more than I would think.

Why doesn't anyone talk about this? She was just a "normal" girl loving life like anyone else her age! Why did this happen? I will never understand, but if anything, I now know how fragile the brain can be. It's so important to see the warning signs in your loved ones.

The episode lasted about four weeks until she started to come out of it with the help of therapy and medications. Bailey spent three years in an incredible program full of support while she continued to work and go back to school. She got through it, and the diagnosis is still out there that that she may have bipolar disorder. One doctor didn't believe she has it because she believes the depression is what caused the episode, yet the other doctor believes this is her diagnosis.

Whatever she has it doesn't matter. All that matters to me is that she is well and that she should never feel afraid or ashamed to talk about it.

Depression, psychosis, mental health disorders have no face. They can happen to ANYONE just like it happened to my beautiful, successful, full-of-life daughter.

I look back now and sometimes still can't believe this was reality, but it was, and it made all of us stronger and educated in something so unknown. I want to be a source for anyone who needs advice or support, as it's so scary to witness this as a parent.

Since this happened, Bailey has changed but for the better. She is aware now of what happened and open and honest about her experience as she sees it. She wants nothing more than to be able to help another person not feel so alone.

Not everyone has the support she had, and it's scary to go through this and even scarier to share what she experienced. I am so proud of my daughter. She is a young girl like everyone else who loves her family, friends, Starbucks, shopping, making people laugh, writing, and her art.

I am so incredibly proud of her for being so open about her experience and wanting to change the life of just one other person if she can. If I can give one bit of advice, it would be to really listen to your child when they say they are struggling. I just thought it was normal to have all these feelings when going to a new school and being away from home. A part of me feels so much guilt for not doing more until it was almost too late…but I really didn't know what was happening!

I honestly thought it would get better. I could write my own book on this entire experience, but for now, this is the short form. Be there for your loved ones and help stop the stigma on mental health.

I could have lost my beautiful daughter due to depression, and I am so forever grateful for her; she inspires me so much! She went through one of the most difficult things I have witnessed, and she picked up and made her life even better.

Dad – Carlos Telo

I'll start by saying this; I wish I knew then what I know now. You see, until this happened to my daughter Bailey, I knew very little about mental illness and what it does to an individual.

Bailey was an intelligent kid that walked around with a quiet confidence. She always had big dreams and aspirations. On the day she had her psychosis episode, I was scared, shocked, and just wished it would stop. My immediate thought was, is she on drugs?

As time went on it was clear to her mother and I that this was not the outcome of drug use, but what we later found out would be a manic psychosis episode. Bailey found the help she needed with a psychosis program in our city and continued to use the tools she learned to become a smart, confident adult living with a mental illness.

It's funny; Bailey often tells me that I am her hero for surviving cancer, but what she doesn't know is that she is also mine.

It takes a very strong person to not only overcome but live with mental illness. I have no doubt in my mind that Bailey will fulfill all her hopes and dreams, going into adulthood and live a fulfilling life.

Aunt - Charlene Stavro

I have never seen anything like this in my lifetime, and I hope I never see it again. I did not think in my wildest dreams/nightmares that this could happen. I was totally ignorant about mental illness. As Bailey moved through this, I saw a little girl, and I felt like I needed to wrap my arms around her, protect her, and shield her from the world. No one knew how it would end or if it would. How would this affect her future? Today she is Bailey, always on the go and ready for new adventures. It did not steal her sparkle; I think she shines brighter. To know Bailey is to love her.

Stepmom – Jennifer Telo

I was asked to write a blurb about my beautiful bonus daughters' experience with manic psychosis. To be honest, I don't know where to begin. It feels like a lifetime ago, although it was only a few years ago. I am so proud of her to write her story and let others going through the same know they are not alone. That they can succeed.

It's not easy getting the right help, adjusting, and readjusting medications. I applaud her battle and her courage to be so open and honest with her journey. I'm sure writing about it is somewhat therapeutic and healing, in a way.

It was very scary to watch her go through this. I remember sitting with her in her grandma's house. I took a turn to watch over her. We were all afraid to let her be by herself.

I remember her wanting me to look through her journal. It was covered in drawings, and she talked the whole time at a non-stop, fast pace. She kept relating everything about her to the Friends tv series.

It was hard to watch her in these hyper states. It was even harder to witness her talk about the dead people she would see in these rooms. This was not the same girl I watched grow up.

I wondered, I am sure we all wondered, what did we do to her to make her like this? She was so loved by everyone. I felt like it was all getting to her. A breaking point. She always worked so hard to please everyone. Was it all too much? I couldn't imagine being seventeen and going to university away from home.

The newness, the pressure to get good grades, meeting new people. Did she feel like a failure for wanting to take time off? Did she have guilt for getting in a minor accident with someone in the car? Did she hate the fact that both of her parents now had other children?

In the end, all that mattered was to focus on healing. She got into a wonderful program. We learned so much from her. It was definitely a hard journey, and even after being on medication, you could sometimes tell when she needed meds adjusted. Since she was so open and honest with her medical team, I think they could always tell as well. Although Bailey was always excitable, you could just tell that something wasn't right. She talked a mile a minute, and her goals were a little excessive. Then there were times that she just wanted to sleep.

I know that Bailey is in a good place now. She has learned so much about herself. She has so much ahead of her. As long as she knows she will always have her family on her side, she will go places beyond her own imagination!

Aunt – Jenna Eager

I'm so proud of Bailey for all that she has overcome. Bailey was on Facetime with me the morning of her episode. She was not herself and kept telling me she could see our passing loved ones in her room. I phoned my mom immediately, and right after she called my sister. My sister sped over. It was nothing like I had ever seen before, and I was so worried for her.

What I remember the most was when my mom called me to tell me that she was on her way home. For the next few weeks, I stayed at my moms and watched over Bailey. All of us had shifts throughout the day to ensure that she was not alone.

I specifically remember sleeping with Bailey in her bed almost every night because she was seeing things. She would only fall asleep if I was there. I am so proud of how far she has come. My niece is the most resilient and inspirational girl I have ever met.

Bestie #1 – Maddy Moore

I have never encountered manic psychosis in my life. I have never seen any close friends or family go through what Bailey went through. I won't sugarcoat it; I was worried when my best friends and I visited Bailey one afternoon when she was in a period of manic psychosis.

Of course, I had a ton of questions going through my head when I first saw Bailey. I was so uneducated on her mental illness. What triggered her behaviour? What can I do to help? How long does manic psychosis last?

Fast forward a couple of years, and I can say I am so proud of Bailey's resilience. She lights up any room she enters and knows how to make everyone laugh. I am also so proud of Bailey to have written this book! She is able to share her story with people who are not educated on these topics, like myself or for those going through something like Bailey. I hope she inspires readers just like she inspires me every day to learn more about mental illnesses. She makes the best out of every situation and can just laugh it out!

Bestie #2 – Lindsay Puls

As Bailey's former roommate and someone who still lives close to her in our hometown, I firsthand witnessed a lot of her struggles while dealing with manic psychosis.

Unfortunately, I have a lot of stories where I saw Bailey battle with her mental health, but I will be brief and share one which I think really encapsulates Bailey for the amazing, strong person she is.

Bailey and I both applied and got the really cool opportunity to be on a student committee that helps plan Orientation Week for first years. At the end of the summer, around August, we had to spend almost a week on campus to start preparing for the events of Frosh Week. Flashback to a few weeks earlier, Bailey is in the middle of manic psychosis, a scary time for all of us but especially for her.

Despite this, Bailey didn't default on her responsibilities of this committee and decided to join me for the week in Waterloo. Not only did she fulfill her responsibilities, she OWNED this week.

Bailey couldn't drink due to starting new meds but still joined for the drinking nights, got herself some Kool-Aids, and cracked the funniest jokes about it all night. Despite still having irregular, bad sleeps, she was incredibly positive every day and energized the entire group. Bailey also made friends with probably every single student there (which was hundreds), making a meaningful connection with all of them. She truly made this week so much better for everyone, especially me, as I was very glad to have time with my bestie.

I think back on this story very fondly. It is a perfect example of owning who you are and embracing your flaws, and like Bailey, turning them into something beautiful, lighthearted, and even funny!

Despite being in the midst of manic psychosis, Bailey still brought incredible levity and humor to any situation, not to mention was also the life of the party. Her tenacity and resilience inspire me, and I'm so proud to call her my best friend!

Bestie #3 – Alana Hitsman

Bailey and I have been best friends for as long as I can remember. I love her so much, and I am so grateful to have her in my life. Watching Bailey experience her manic episode was very traumatic and unlike anything I have ever experienced before.

Our friend group was concerned for Bailey because we greatly admire and care for her so much. We all just wanted to do whatever we could to help her in any way possible. I am so proud of Bailey and all that she has overcome. She is such an amazing human, and I am so lucky to be able to call her my best friend.

Bestie #4 – Sophie Radake

Seeing your best friend and someone you love in a state of manic psychosis is not something that should be taken lightly. Seeing Bailey this way was unlike anything I had experienced before; it was scary and confusing all at the same time. I often wondered what would happen next and how I could best help Bailey.

I know Bailey's story will inspire many and help anyone who may be going through the same thing, whether you are personally experiencing manic psychosis or you have a loved one who is. I am grateful to be able to watch Bailey flourish into the person she is today and who she continues to be.

Bailey, thanks for always being a light in everyone's lives. You are courageous, brave, and inspiring. I can't wait to watch you accomplish so many more great things.

Bestie #5 – Devyn Maybee

It's hard to not place blame on yourself for failing to recognize the signs of your best friend experiencing a manic episode.

I lived with Bailey in first-year university which was one of the hardest years of both our lives. I often felt guilty for trying to force Bailey out of our apartment and experience the "university culture" because I knew she didn't want to. Conversely, I also knew it wasn't right to just leave her in her room to cry herself to sleep every night.

Needless to say, I was trying to "fix" her and felt that it was my responsibility to do so. I know now, however, that it wasn't. My only responsibility as her roommate and friend was to simply be there for her and to listen to her feelings.

A year later when Bailey finally made the difficult, yet mature decision to drop out of school, I honestly felt like it was my fault –not that she dropped out, but that she stayed so much longer than she should have. I was devastated, of course, but knew this was what Bailey needed to help herself heal.

Then came her manic episode. Frankly, I wasn't shocked that this was happening to her because it just gave us the answers we were longing for and made everything make sense.

I still remember the first time I visited her in the summer; I brought her two of her favourite things; a journal (which you all now know of as "the book"), and an iced coffee. As I handed Bailey her go-to Starbucks order, she frowned and said, "I can't drink coffee". That's when it hit me, just how serious this situation was. It's crazy when your normal routine gets knocked down and you witness your friend fail to do or enjoy the simple pleasures of life that she once could.

That summer, I was working a job three hours away, but I drove down to visit her almost every week. I knew that was what Bailey needed the most–just a small slice of normal. I hope I was able to provide that for her because if it was me in that situation, which it has been as of late, I knew she would and does the same.

I don't think Bailey realizes the impact she has on her people. Her energy is infectious, and laugh is contagious. She exudes a powerful, yet quiet confidence and is 100% unapologetically herself. Intelligent, courageous, ambitious, and loyal…I could go on forever.

Most importantly, Bailey is an empath. She uses her experience to connect with others and make them feel that they are never alone. I am so lucky and extremely grateful to have experienced her impact, firsthand.

There are so many lessons I can take away from not only witnessing a friend's manic psychosis episode but also from just being someone's friend.

Here are just a few:

1. You can't fix or save people. All you can do is be there for them when they need you the most.

2. Friendships are almost never 50/50, and they should most definitely not hold the expectation of a

transaction. Sometimes one person will carry 90% of the relationship and if you are doing it out of the selflessness of your heart, it's okay.

3. Mental health is challenging, and you never know when someone is going to get better. It can take a long time. So, stay with them. It's much easier for someone to give up on themselves if everyone else around them has too.

4. Mental illness doesn't just affect the individual going through it but also the people around them. This is not to place a burden on the person experiencing pain but to exhibit just how important community can be in a time of need. Grieving the person, they once were and

learning to understand and accept the person they are becoming

5. Finally, a mental health diagnosis is not a bad thing. It is simply just information about yourself that you can use to adapt and hopefully, one day heal.

Colleague – Kristi Kearns

I remember watching Bailey at the time, envious of her seemingly boundless energy and yet concerned that she could never seem to slow down.

Bailey spoke fast, she moved fast, and there was no stopping her. I tried to advocate for her at work, my instincts telling me she was not okay, but not having the knowledge to recognize what was coming and feeling powerless to help her.

Watching her journey has helped me as I struggled to help my daughter as she went through her own battle with mental health.

It is a lonely place to stand, hopeless, powerless, and despairing that it will get better for your child. I know now that it will, it does, but it requires patience, compassion, dedication...and a little Mama Bear anger somedays.

Non-biological sister – Hayley Morgan

It's difficult to understand mental health and all it encompasses.

As someone who grew up in a generation with a stigma attached to it, it's a relief that brave people like Bailey have brought more awareness and visibility to the subject.

With all of the progress society has made surrounding mental health, there is still so much more work to be done, which is why I am so very proud of and inspired by Bailey. Offering vulnerability to speak to her experiences in such a public manner is the definition of bravery.

I was present during this time in Bailey's life, yet what I saw only scratched the surface of what was truly going on. I'd never understood what the meaning of "going manic" truly meant and never fathomed there was a state in which hallucinations were involved.

I remember getting phone calls from her loved ones asking if I had any insight into what was going on because of how out of character her behavior was. In hindsight, I was being asked to confirm if she'd suffered an injury or if there was any known drug use.

It's alarming to think that those alternatives were easier to digest than what was actually happening.

Thankfully, Bailey was able to get the diagnosis and began getting the help she needed. I've maintained a great relationship with Bailey to this day. Watching her grow as a person from this experience has been truly inspiring. It's still hard to wrap my brain around what she went through, but it hasn't stopped her from being authentically herself.

It makes perfect sense that Bailey has decided to write about her experiences as she has a true desire to help others. That can be seen in her day-to-day life. I can't wait to witness even more of this amazing person, and the impact this book will have on her life and the lives of people who have gone through something similar.

Bailey; you're such an intelligent, charismatic, beautiful person. You shine brighter than most and your talent is limitless.

Non-biological sister – Mara Connacher

It is never easy watching someone you love struggle, especially when that person doesn't understand what they are going through.

You're watching this person you know to be so full of positivity and literally the definition of a bright light and shining star, behave in a way that isn't who you know them to be.

As someone with their own past with the dark side of mental illness, I wanted to support Bailey in any way I could. Being understanding, kind, and non-judgmental. I didn't want her to feel alone as so many of us do in our battles with mental illness.

Watching Bailey navigate through this journey and come out the other side has been so inspiring; actually, it's bigger than that I just can't find a word for it. Bailey is a one-of-a-kind amazing person, full of

confidence, drive, positivity, and vulnerability. I feel

extremely fortunate to have this ray of light in my life!

A ROUGH PATCH

Healing from this baby car accident, a wild manic episode, and being a university dropout took a whole lot of energy out of me. I'm proud of myself for accepting that I needed a lot of help, and still do!

As I mentioned before, I was in an early intervention psychosis program at a hospital in my city. As I write today, it is January 25th, 2023.

I graduated from the 3-year psychosis program in the summer of 2022. It took a lot of hard work, time, medication switches, and everything else in between. I'm feeling the best I've felt in a while. I'm finally so excited to have my story out there! I still attend monthly appointments with my psychiatrist to discuss

my medication. My brain is healing, and so is my heart.

GETTING HELP

Getting help is something that I didn't think I would ever need. After my manic episode, I knew this wasn't just an option anymore.

I had therapists in university who I dreaded seeing. It wasn't them; it was me. They were great therapists who were trying to help, but I was stubborn and didn't want to put the work in.

I felt like therapy was pointless, and my mind was set on the fact that it would never help. Why would talking to somebody else help me when I would much rather just lay in bed all day and watch YouTube videos. I thought that I would feel like this forever. I thought I would always feel numb.

To be completely honest, I like to think of myself as a living, walking, and breathing example of "it does get better".

It usually won't happen immediately, and it could take months or even years. Everyone's different though. Just think about it this way; you've already just dealt with your darkest days, so chances are it'll only get better from here. Remember that when you feel hopeless.

Therapy is now something that I find so much value in. I started it because I didn't have much choice after the episode. I'm glad I did though. I met some of the best individuals. It's cool because your therapist most likely doesn't know you outside their office. In my opinion, it's easy to talk to people who are outsiders.

While we're on this tangent, there's many different types of therapy. You can do one-on-one, group therapy, cognitive behavioral therapy…the opportunities are endless.

To me, therapy is like gold. Make it a habit to do something for yourself, even if it's just a simple self-care routine. Self-care doesn't necessarily have to be booking a vacation or getting a cosmetic procedure.

Self-care can also be grabbing a coffee, meeting with a friend, or maybe purchasing that necklace you've always seen but never bought.

Do something that will help you! I'm all for self-care. You'll feel your best when you start finding the joy in little things and continue to take care of yourself. You've probably heard that before but believe

it this time!

DAILY LOGS

I kept my own daily/monthly logs during all of my mental health challenges. It's interesting to look back and see how far I've come.

August 23, 2019:

If you were to ask me how I'm feeling now, I would say great! It has been almost a month since I faced extreme trauma and hallucinations. I'm feeling a lot like myself again. Don't even ask me about the journal I wrote during that time. I'll never publish that one. Like I said before, I wrote it backwards, so it will probably only make sense to me. **Present me:** My grandma, Char, and I were talking about this recently. They told me that when they tried to read it, nothing clicked. Everything I wrote made sense to me, as I was in a manic state. I tried to read my journal the other day and didn't understand a thing. Shocker.

That journal is something that I'll probably never open again. I don't ever want to be in that state of mind again. Manic psychosis is a scary illness. I even transferred it all into a new book so that it was not written backwards. Yeah, don't ask. When I bring up "THE BOOK" to my family, they usually get a little bit frightened when I take it out.

Anyways, I'm back, and I'm feeling a lot better. I've had the opportunity to return to work and hang out with friends and family. This has been so helpful for me. I've been studying neuroscience because I want to understand what's happening in my brain. My grandma thinks it's cool. Alright, well…I'm still healing but I'm a lot better than I was a month ago. Signing off.

November 13, 2019:

Today I dropped out of school. I have no words. I don't even know how to feel. My mom came up to school today to help me unenroll myself and speak with a guidance counselor.

I'm almost embarrassed because I couldn't handle this. All my friends could. I know I shouldn't compare myself to others, but I can't help it. They were able to stick it out.

Why couldn't I? I feel absolutely defeated. Who knows what will happen next. I'm trying my best to be optimistic.

November 20, 2019:

I'm back at work now part-time. I love everyone I work with, with all my heart, but I honestly don't feel like myself. I feel like my coworkers may be noticing how miserable I am. I honestly don't know how to cover it up. I'm super depressed, but I'm trying not to show it.

Dec 25, 2019:

I thought I would be happier this Christmas because I don't have school to worry about. I'm not. I'm still beating myself up since I dropped out. It sucks that I'm continually feeling like this.

April 9, 2020:

My mental health has been relatively poor the last couple of months. This worldwide pandemic has flipped everybody's world upside down, including my own. My days consist of constantly lying-in bed. I feel numb.

June 11, 2020:

The weather has gotten nicer, which has really lifted my mood. I'm starting to feel a lot like myself again. Maybe the meds are doing their job after all. My days consist of lying out by the pool, watching the clouds pass, and having lovely conversations with friends that come by.

July 20, 2020:

I'm finally back at work! My first day back was great, although the new protocol has made it much different! I missed my coworkers so much, and I'm thankful to have reunited with them once again. They make me the happiest girl in the world.

September 9, 2020:

OMG! I'm starting school today! I'm both nervous and excited. Ps. This whole zoom thing is weird. This is definitely something I'll have to get used to.

November 13, 2020:

I'm finally the happiest that I've felt in a while! I have discovered a lot of my interests. I love the journalism program I'm taking; it's seriously so much fun! I've met incredible people and professors! Work is going great too! We're out of lockdown, and I'm able to see my amazing coworkers throughout the week!

I've been spending more time with friends and family and feel 110% like myself again. If you were to ask me how I was this time last year, I would describe myself in three words; depressed, alone, and defeated. Now I can say that I feel ecstatic, relieved, and free.

December 10, 2020:

Hypomania: Yeah, didn't see this one coming. The state I have been in within the last couple of weeks has been pretty elevated. I've been super happy and energetic, but maybe too elevated.

I went to my monthly appointment and spoke to my therapists and psychiatrists about how I was feeling. I mentioned my high energy levels. My high energy turned into what's classified as hypomania. This is one of the early stages of psychosis.

To prevent psychosis from happening again, I need to do something that scares me. I must go on the medication I was on when I first dealt with psychosis. Honestly, I'm not too fond of this medication. It made me gain a lot of weight the first time, but it works. The first night that I took the medication, it knocked me

out. It's meant to slow down the brain. I felt drowsy
for a few days.

December 28, 2020:

I've begun to tolerate the psychosis medication, and
I'm getting used to it. I am, however, trying to watch
what I eat more carefully. It's working, so that's all that
matters, I guess.

January 7, 2021:

New year, same me. I've been recommended a new
medication that essentially does the same thing as my
last one. It doesn't increase my appetite.

January 3, 2022:

Woah. Long-time no talk. To be honest, I forgot about
this book. I was losing motivation. Lots has happened
this year. I will be beginning my last semester of my
college program! I have been working hard at finding

internships, looking more into my career, and exploring options. I set some new year's resolutions for myself:

1. Maintain healthy relationships with others

2. Check up on loved ones

3. Drink lots of water

4. Move my body

It's crazy how so much can change in a year. I feel mature and ready to confidently start a new chapter in my life. I am proud of myself. I've been through a long and challenging mental health journey, that's for sure…but it has made me so strong. I want nothing more in life than to help the people around me. Mental health is hard to deal with, and you're not alone. There's almost always a light at the end of the tunnel. Remember those words when life feels impossible.

January 30, 2023: <3

So much has happened in my life! I travelled to Greece in September with my best friends, graduated from college, and took a lot of time to work on myself.

I'm the happiest I've been in a very long time! I'm just about done writing this book! I'm over the moon, and I can't wait to get my story out there in hopes to help others. I finally feel free! I know it sounds cringey, but one of my biggest dreams is coming true; finally!

As a little kid I knew that I wanted to write a book or illustrate one. Although what happened to me was terrifying, it gave me the opportunity to write this book and chase my dreams. Priceless.

Journaling is one of my favourite coping mechanisms by far. I also love stationary shopping and buying cute little pens and notebooks!

Even though I've healed, I still have bad days. If something upsets me during my day, I reflect on it at night. I'll write about everything before I go to bed, shut the book, and never look at it again.

Closing the book is my way of removing those negative thoughts from my life. I do this when I'm stressed, except I'll go back and reference what I wrote when the week is over.

If I know I'm going to have a stressful week, I'll start writing what I must accomplish on Monday.

As the days go on, I'll write about what happened or the things that are stressing me out.

On Friday, I'll reread the journal starting with Monday. I love this part because then I can see what I have accomplished. Even if I accomplished nothing, I still give myself a pat on the back for writing about my feelings.

Buy yourself a cute journal, some fun pens, and get going. Journaling is a healthy way to deal with your thoughts, and it has helped me so much! Make it a habit to stay consistent with it. Hold yourself accountable and tell yourself that you will journal either in the morning or at night. I promise it's worth it!

YOUR DAILY LOGS
119

Write how you're doing in this section. It could be what you're thankful for, something you're sad or happy about, something cool you did, or whatever you're feeling! Putting your thoughts down on paper can help you piece those ideas together visually. In my opinion, it can also be very therapeutic. I love to reflect before I go to bed. I find that it really helps me! You're the only one who is in control of YOU! :)

____

____

____

____

____

____

____

____

RESOURCES FOR HELP

Kids Help Phone – Online, telephone, one-on-one support (text messaging), tailored to youth in Canada. Their website provides access to others' stories, activities to build personal skills & a directory that shows helpful support programs near you.

Good2talk – Provides service for post-secondary students (Ontario & Nova Scotia)
- Ontario Support:
    - 1-866-925-5454
    - Text GOOD2TALKON to 686868

Wellness Together Canada – Created due to the increase of mental health and substance use difficulties following the pandemic.
- For all ages
- Over-the-phone counselling
    - 1-866-585-0445 (adults)
    - 1-888-668-6810 (youth)

CAMH – The Centre for Addiction & Mental Health
- Known to be Canada's largest facility for addictions and mental health
- Wide variety of services
- Help with services:
    - 416-535-8501: Option 2
- Mental Illness & Addiction Index
    - Helpful resource to educate yourself on mental health related terms, signs, symptoms, and more.

CONCLUSION

If you made it this far, thank you. Truly, from the bottom of my heart. I hope that my story could help you or someone else in your life.

My biggest piece of advice is to never be ashamed of what you're going through. We all have something going on – big or small. Recognizing that you may need help is a good thing! It's never too late to make changes or heal.

If I'm in a good headspace and feeling my best mentally, everything else will be a breeze. Take care of yourself, listen to your body, and when in doubt take three deep breaths. A close friend of mine taught me

that. ♡

REFERENCES

The Centre for Addiction and Mental Health. (2023).
    Retrieved February 2023, from
    https://www.camh.ca

Gibson, T. (2023). *Tyrese Gibson quote: "You will always
    grow through – what you go through.".* Quotefancy.
    Retrieved March 6, 2023, from
    https://quotefancy.com/quote/1681441/Tyres
    e-Gibson-You-will-always-grow-through-what-
    you-go-through

Good2Talk. (2023, March). Retrieved March 6, 2023,
    from https://good2talk.ca/

Kids Help Phone. (2023, March). Retrieved March 6,
    2023, from https://kidshelpphone.ca/

Psychosis. CAMH. (2023). Retrieved March 6, 2023,
    from https://www.camh.ca/en/health-
    info/mental-illness-and-addiction-
    index/psychosis

Wellness Together Canada. (2022). Retrieved
    February 2023, from
    https://www.wellnesstogether.ca/en-CA

Fin

ABOUT THE AUTHOR

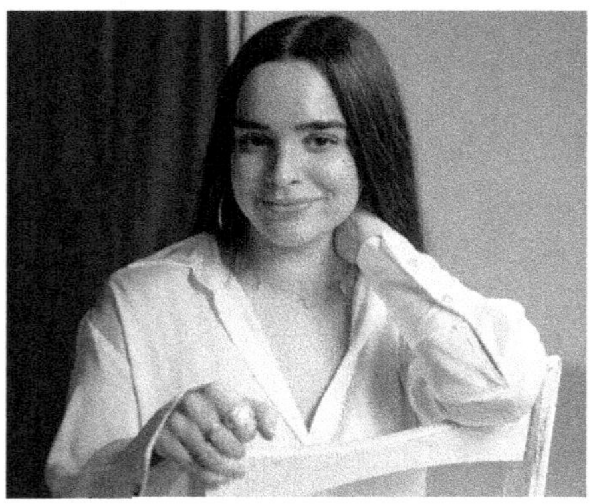

Photo by: Joanna Roselli

Bailey Emily is a 22-year-old girl with a whole bunch of interests. She has a college diploma in journalism and has always been focused on her writing. Bailey grew up as a competitive dancer and enjoyed anything she could get creative with. She loves life chats, deep breaths, journaling, and dreaming about becoming a well-known book writer/illustrator. She hopes her story will reach many people who may be struggling in silence.

Be yourself, love hard, and have fun.

It costs nothing to be kind.

9 781738 952311